# NO MORE WRINKLES
# by Tova

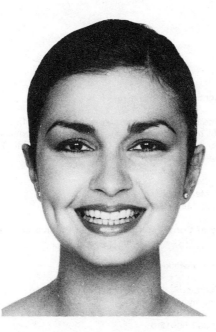

## A PERIGEE BOOK

Perigee Books
are published by
G. P. Putnam's Sons
200 Madison Avenue
New York, NY 10016

Inside photos: Torkil Gudnason
Stylist: Mark Mussler
Drawings: Maria Burgaleta

**Library of Congress Cataloging in Publication Data**

Tova.
  No more wrinkles.

  1. Exercise.   2. Facial muscles.   3. Face—
Care and hygiene.   4. Skin—Wrinkles.   I. Title.
RA781.T68   1981      646.7′2      80-39546
ISBN 0-399-50515-6

First Perigee Printing, 1981
PRINTED IN THE UNITED STATES OF AMERICA

# Introduction

There's never a good time to discover new wrinkles on your face. Somehow they always seem to appear just when you think you've gotten it all together. Your makeup is just right; you like the way your hair looks; you think you've finally learned to dress smartly in a way that reflects your personality. And then, there it is—a creeping crow's-foot at the edge of your eye, fine accordion pleating across your upper lip, a permanent furrow in the middle of your brow, or worse, those awful first cross-hatchings over your cheek. These lines date you, and they don't fit in with the image you have of yourself. Your mind's eye remembers someone else, a younger, fresher you.

These wrinkles and furrows seem out of place. Yes, you've been told they're inevitable, but somehow they don't belong on your face. They weren't there yesterday, and you dread to think what you will find when you look tomorrow.

Well, there's a good chance your thinking is right. The real you may be smoother and younger-looking than the face you now see. Those wrinkles may very likely not belong on your face—at least not yet. And, you *can* do something about it with a little time and effort.

Although skin does wrinkle and sag with age as it loses elasticity and the tissues begin to break down, there are many other factors over which you *do* have control that are far more critical than age in causing premature wrinkling of the skin. Your most important enemies are neglect and ignorance. I can provide you with what you should know and do, but then you have to act if you want to win the battle against the clock.

Learn to recognize your enemies so you can fight them on their own ground. Think of these culprits as the Sinister Seven:

1. The Scourge of the Sun
2. Dehydration
3. Dos and Don'ts of Dieting and Your Diet
4. Smoking and Other Bad Habits
5. Stress
6. Gravity
7. Loss of Muscle Tone

First we will run through this list of enemies so that you will know how to prevent premature wrinkling of the skin. Then I will give you my exercise plan, developed specifically to tone and tighten the face. Together the knowledge and the exercises can teach you how to keep your skin and face as fresh and youthful-looking as nature will allow.

# THE SINISTER SEVEN

## 1. The Scourge of the Sun

If you spend a good deal of your leisure time in the warm weather soaking up the sun's rays, don't be surprised if your face ends up looking like a dried-up prune. The ultraviolet rays of the sun—the same wavelengths that cause you to tan and give you a burn if you're not careful—actually break down the connective tissues under the skin, causing damage that becomes irreparable over the course of time. The fine web of connective tissue supporting your skin and holding it in place is made up primarily of the proteins collagen and elastin. These fibers are what give young skin its characteristic smoothness, suppleness, and elasticity. Exposure to the sun literally destroys the collagen and causes the elastin to increase in thick, brittle clumps. This produces skin that is dry, inelastic, and that wrinkles easily. Aging alone, with no exposure to the sun, will effect a slight decrease in the amount of elastin; the collagen will become a bit thin and fibrous but will remain relatively the same.

With this knowledge, dermatologists have agreed conclusively that repeated exposure to the sun is a far more important factor than chronological age in causing premature wrinkling of the skin. Dr. John F. Romano, attending dermatologist at New York Hospital-Cornell Medical Center, told me that if you took a sample of skin from an unexposed part of the body—say the buttocks—of a fifty-year-old person and compared it under a microscope with a similar sample from a twenty-year-old, you probably couldn't tell which was which. Skin from the face of a twenty-year-old Floridian who sunbathed regularly, however, might well be mistaken for the skin of an old person.

Sun damage, which doctors refer to as solar elastosis, takes years to appear, and it is irreversible. If you've insisted on deep tanning every summer, all you can do at this point with your newfound knowledge is prevent further damage. If you've never been a sun-worshiper, you are in a lucky minority. The first lesson you must learn to ensure no more wrinkles is simple: *Avoid exposure to the sun.*

Since most of us are not about to give up the pleasure of the beach entirely or throw away our tennis rackets and golf clubs, it is nice to know that in recent years, very good protective sunscreens have been developed. A number of effective chemicals have been approved by the U.S. Food and Drug Administration. One of the best known is PABA (para-amino benzoic acid). In compound with alcohol in lotions, creams, and gels, it is applied to the skin, where it absorbs many of the sun's dangerous ultraviolet rays before they can reach your body.

Depending on how effective they are in blocking the sun, these sunscreens are usually rated with an SPF (Sun Protection Factor) number that ranges anywhere from 2 to 15. The lower the number, the less protection and the less time you can spend in the sun without burning. A rating of 15 indicates maximum protection, which with proper use will prevent most tanning as well as burning. Dr. Romano usually recommends an SPF of 8 to 10 for many of his patients with normal skin. This allows slow tanning, while affording considerable protection.

## 2. Dehydration

When moisture is lost from the skin, the dessicated tissue shrivels up and wrinkles. Even young skin can look old and tired when it is dehydrated. Luckily, dryness is often easy to avoid. True, some natural dryness comes with age, as our hormones change and the glands in our skin reduce their secretions. But by far the worst causes of dryness are environmental. Therefore you must learn to protect yourself properly from the elements.

The sun, of course, remains your worst enemy. Always use a moisturizer, even under your sunscreen. Heat alone will cause evaporation that will deplete the moisture in your skin. If you sunbathe and you do burn, your damaged skin is going to become dry, itchy, and scaly. The pain from a sunburn takes anywhere from 2 to 16 hours to develop fully. Don't wait for it to set in. If your skin is red, treat it as soon as you get home. Shower or bathe in cool to tepid water, washing carefully with a gentle soap, such as castile. Do not use a deodorant soap; the chemicals will only aggravate your condition. Towel off gently, patting rather than rubbing your skin. Dry yourself only enough to remove excessive moisture, but try to leave a slight layer of dampness on your skin. Then apply a rich moisturizer all over your body. A urea-based cream or ointment is best. This will help your skin to absorb water. Lotions, which are mostly water themselves, tend to be too thin to be really helpful in sealing in moisture. The water locked under a heavier moisturizer will be absorbed by your skin, which will ease the dryness and help prevent wrinkling. If you have any difficulty in choosing a moisturizer, either because you have hypoallergenic skin or because you don't like the odor of a urea-based product, you might want to consult a professional dermatologist, who can recommend the best choice for your particular type of skin.

If it's not the summer sun that's attacking your skin, chances are it's the ravages of winter. Dry heat and blustery winds can take the moisture right out of your skin's delicate cells, leaving them shriveled and scaly. In winter, use a humidifier to regulate your environment. Makeup, applied over a good moisturizer, will act as a protective screen from the elements. And always shield your face with a moisturizer when you are not wearing makeup, especially at night. Remember, it is always preferable to apply moisturizer over slightly damp rather than bone-dry skin. If you have a problem with wrinkling around the eyes, you might want to invest in an eye cream, which is simply a moisturizer with a heavier oil base to seal in the fluids.

Hydration, or water absorption, is the basic principle behind most of those "miracle" wrinkle creams being marketed by many cosmetic companies these days. Such creams have no magic rejuvenating effect on the nucleus of the skin cells. But they do facilitate the absorption of moisture into the stratum corneum, the outermost layer of the epidermis. This layer is made up of dry dead and dying cells, which rise to the surface of the skin before being sloughed off. All fine lines and wrinkles show up first in this layer of the skin. Pumping these cells full of water causes swelling and smoothing, which erases fine lines and wrinkles temporarily. Some of these creams work very well for 3 to 4 hours at a stretch. For permanent erasure, especially if wrinkles are advanced, plastic surgery is still the only answer.

## 3. Dos and Don'ts of Dieting and Your Diet

Repeated fluctuations in weight, especially if they are extreme, can contribute significantly to premature aging and wrinkling of the skin. If you lose too much weight too quickly, you may dissolve a lot of the fat buoying up the skin without allowing time for new connective tissue to form. The result is a sunken, saggy look that is conducive to wrinkling.

Repeated weight gain and loss may also take some of the elasticity out of the skin, so that it collapses and wrinkles up like crepe paper. Just think of a rubber balloon that is inflated and deflated time after time. Soon it doesn't feel the same anymore. It loses its smoothness and elasticity, until finally, it begins to pucker in wrinkles and break down.

It is healthiest to keep your weight steady, within medically standardized bounds. If you are overweight and you need to lose some pounds, by all means diet, but do so sensibly. Check with a doctor to determine the proper diet for you. Your goal should be to lose weight gradually while you exercise, so that you get maximum benefit from both and your skin has time to repair itself as your body changes.

Especially if you are dieting, be sure you are getting all the nutrients you need. Adequate vitamins A and C and the minerals zinc and iron are particularly important in maintaining beautiful, wrinkle-free skin. Protein for building new tissue and a modicum of fat to permit absorption of the fat-soluble vitamins are also important. And be sure to drink plenty of fluids. Water to flush out your system and keep you hydrated is a marvelous drink, particularly for dieters.

## 4. Smoking and Other Bad Habits

Many experts have noted the connection between smoking and wrinkles. The cause seems to be not some chemical in tobacco, but the physical act of smoking. The contortion of the mouth involved in inhaling and the squinting that often accompanies the act when smoke gets in the eyes, practiced as a regular habit, can etch fine wrinkles around the lips and eyes.

The same is true of any habitual idiosyncratic expression—chewing your lip, wrinkling your nose, pulling at your skin, resting your cheek on your hand to support your head. They all contort your face and pull at the tissues, eventually stretching the skin so that it sags and wrinkles.

The reason this happens is that the skin on the face is less tightly bound to the muscles below it than elsewhere on the body. The connective tissues are fragile and need all the help they can get.

The best way to avoid these types of unnecessary wrinkles is to make a list of all the bad facial habits and idiosyncratic expressions you are aware of. Ask a close friend if he or she has noticed any others. Concentrate on developing an awareness of how you hold your face so that you catch yourself every time you scrunch up your nose or start picking at your skin. And if you smoke, the choice is yours—beauty or butts.

# 5. Stress

Stress is probably the greatest silent ravager of the human body. One of the obvious places it shows its damage is on the skin of the face. With some people, you can chart the course of their daily lives by the condition of their complexion. For some the toll is blemishes; for others, such problems as eczema and psoriasis. And for many of us, it's those tight little lines around the mouth and eyes, and furrows on the forehead.

We all tend to express our emotions in our facial carriage. How often have you heard: "My, you look like you're in pain!" or "What's wrong? You look as if you've just lost your best friend." Tension contorts our expression, etching fine lines and wrinkles into the face and adding extra twists and folds to otherwise smooth skin.

One prominent doctor told me that there is no doubt in his mind that thinking unhappy or angry thoughts too often can cause "worry lines" and wrinkles, especially in relation to the corrugator muscles. According to *Gray's Anatomy*, the classic medical text, "The Corrugator muscles draw the eyebrow downward and inward, producing the vertical wrinkles of the forehead. It is the frowning muscle, and may be regarded as the principal agent in the expression of suffering."

In addition to making us frown too often, stress can deplete our bodies of some of the vitamins needed for healthy, youthful-looking skin.

Unfortunately, we all have problems that won't go away, and stress is a natural part of life. But there are techniques you can practice to help defuse tension and relieve some of that stress before it strikes your skin. Here are some suggestions:

1. Try to keep things in perspective. When you feel yourself about to explode, ask yourself: Is it worth the aggravation?
2. Try to develop more constructive ways of reacting to stress. If you are late to an important business appointment and there is nothing you can do about it, stop fuming at the traffic; spend the time thinking about what you are going to say at the meeting.
3. Set aside some private time for yourself. This is where the exercises can help. Incorporate them into a 15 to 30 minute "vacation" you give yourself at least every other day. Let it be known that this is *your* time, during which you do not wish to be disturbed. Take a warm bath or lie down with your feet up and listen to some soft music. Do whatever feels right for you. When some of the cares of the day have dropped away and you feel more relaxed and in control, begin your facial exercises. There is nothing like a physical workout to relieve stress and strain. When you are all through, allow an extra 5 or 10 minutes to relax. You'll feel like a new person.

# 6. Gravity

The same force that pulls the tides across the oceans and holds the planets in their orbits acts upon the delicate tissues of your body. Like a perpetually falling drop of water that over eons carves out a hollow in a stone, gravity's slight pull continually tugs at your skin and muscles, causing them to sag toward the ground (think of the droopy little pouches that can appear below the eyes, for example).

Many yoga experts believe that gravity is one of the prime culprits in the aging process. In fact, yoga provides excellent methods for fighting the force of gravity. The inverted (upside-down) postures were specifically designed to counteract the downward pull of gravity on the body. I urge you to investigate a good yoga program in your area. Postures that are particularly effective are the plow, the shoulder stand, and the head stand. These inverted positions also ensure maximum oxygenation of the head and face, which is important for healthy skin.

As a substitute for yoga, you can practice an easy inverted posture simply by lying down on the floor and putting your feet and legs up against a wall. Relax and try to keep your mind blank. Remain in that position for 3 to 5 minutes, until you feel peaceful and calm. When you stand up, be sure to do so slowly.

# 7. Loss of Muscle Tone

Last but not least on the list of skin enemies is poor muscle tone. It is one of the problems you should work most diligently to remedy. When muscles lose their tone, they become soft and flaccid and hang loosely from the bone. On your face this can mean sagging that stretches out the skin and causes wrinkling. Muscle tone diminishes slowly with age, but it falls off sharply with disuse. That is why facial exercises can make an important difference in preserving it.

Good muscle tone is so important, in fact, that at least one prominent plastic surgeon that I know of, Dr. Ivo Janecka of Presbyterian Hospital in New York, recommends facial exercises to most of his patients *before* they enter the hospital for surgical face-lifting. His feeling is that the loose, sagging skin about to be lifted may be dragging down the muscles. When that weight is removed, he wants the muscles underneath to be as tight and firm as possible. This will allow maximum benefit from the facelift and prevent premature stretching and wrinkling of the newly smoothed skin.

Some people wonder why exercises are necessary. After all, your face is always in motion—whether you are talking, laughing, eating, or crying. It gets a workout every day.

You do use some of your facial muscles in your day-to-day life, but probably not all of them. If you're like most people, chances are you tend to chew your food mostly on one side. Do you always enunciate with great clarity, or do you sometimes mumble and slur your words? Perhaps you speak with a regional accent. Some people smile a lot, others tend to frown. You may be developing muscles, unconsciously, in ways that aren't helping you to look your best.

The muscles of the human body are highly specific, and those of the face are no exception. If you chew your food on the right side of your mouth all the time, the muscles of mastication on the left side are not going to become equally well developed. For maximum benefit, each muscle must be exercised individually. My exercise program, which follows, is designed to do just that.

# The Exercise Plan

The following series of 25 exercises is designed to give the facial muscles a vigorous workout. The exercises are simple to perform, and the accompanying photographs and line drawings should make them easy to follow. Most of the movements are not strenuous, but when you finish, your face will certainly feel well used.

As with any physical activity, consult your doctor before beginning a new exercise program. If you have had facial surgery recently, do nothing without checking with your physician. For most people, this program is simple and safe.

These exercises were developed to tone and tighten the facial muscles, to prevent sagging and premature wrinkling. Practiced regularly over a period of time, there should also be some muscle development as well. Since the muscles of the face are very thin, growth will be minimal, but in some areas, the added tissue may be just enough to smooth out fine lines and wrinkles in the outer layer of the skin.

To tone the muscles, you must practice the exercises as described for 10 to 15 minutes at least 3 or 4 days a week. To develop the muscles, you should exercise every day, with increasing repetitions. For most purposes, a gradual increase to 6 or 7 repetitions will be sufficient. For problem spots, a second short session of specific exercises is recommended.

For the most effective results, be sure to follow the instructions carefully. A mirror is a great help, and should be used whenever possible. Don't push yourself at first. Getting into shape takes time. If any pain or discomfort occurs, stop exercising; if it continues, see your doctor.

Exercising your face is good for you—for your looks and for the way you feel. It should be an enjoyable experience as well. Try to set aside a special time for these exercises—and for yourself—each day. Before starting, cleanse your face gently (but do not apply a moisturizer until you are finished). Then lie down with your feet up. Wrap your face in a warm—not hot—towel with an opening for your nose to breathe. Relax and enjoy the peace for at least 3 minutes. Then hold this book in front of your mirror and begin to find the prettier you with *No More Wrinkles*.

# THE CHIN SYNDROME

Nothing gives it away more than a loose, sagging chin. Whether you are old enough to be losing tone or have developed a double chin prematurely, the damage from this syndrome is similar. Because of the slinglike way the muscles of your neck and chin attach to your head, that heavy, flaccid flesh underneath can drag down your whole face.

Luckily, your chin and neck contain relatively large muscles that are easy to work with. The exercises that follow are specifically geared to tone and tighten and to help prevent loss of definition below the face. By firming up underneath, you will relieve some of the pressure on your other facial muscles, pressure that can cause sagging and wrinkling of the skin.

If you are suffering from the Chin Syndrome, chances are you can also afford to shed a few pounds. Check with your doctor, and if he or she says it's ok, put yourself on a sensible, calorically reduced diet, with a goal of losing six pounds in two months. Compared to crash diet programs, this may sound like very slow progress, but medically speaking, the healthiest, most efficient way to lose weight is gradually. By taking your time, you will lose all fat, rather than a combination of fat and healthy muscle tissue, and you will keep the weight off afterward. As you've probably noticed, crash dieters often put the weight they've lost right back on as soon as they stop dieting.

At the end of two months, reevaluate your image. In particular, examine your chin and decide whether or not you need to repeat the program to take off more weight.

At the same time that you are dieting sensibly, be sure to practice your daily exercises. Diet and exercise are always most effective when practiced in combination. If you suffer from the Chin Syndrome, give yourself an extra 5- or 10-minute session to repeat Exercises 1 through 6 and Exercise 22. If you find that you need extra work for a special problem area, do your regular exercise routine when you wake up in the morning; then create your own spot-problem routine with the appropriate exercises and practice it around five o'clock or just before you go to bed. If it's better for your schedule, do your special program in the morning: The point is to exercise regularly.

Remember, don't force any of the exercises. Do them to the best of your ability without straining or allowing yourself to feel any pain or discomfort. You will gradually work up to a full range of muscle use without any unnecessary strain on the tissues.

## 1. Push It Away

It takes extra stress on a muscle to tighten or develop it. We open and close our mouths thousands of times each day, as we talk, eat, yawn, breathe. To put some extra work into opening that lower jaw and attempting to tone the muscles under the chin, this exercise uses your own hand to create resistance against which your muscles have to push. This is a progressive resistance type of exercise.

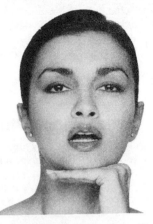

Place the back of your hand flat under your chin. Now try to open your mouth slowly by pushing your lower jaw down. As your mouth opens, push upward with your hand, so that your jaw has to work hard to open your mouth all the way. Repeat 2 more times.

After you have exercised for 2 or 3 weeks, you can work harder with this exercise both by increasing the number of repetitions gradually and by increasing the upward pressure—or resistance—of your hand.

## 2. Squeeze It Away

Your mirror will really help you with this exercise at first. Once you've mastered it, of course, you can practice it anywhere. The more repetitions you build up to, the better. This is a marvelous contraction for the platysma, the large sheet of muscle that covers the neck and chin.

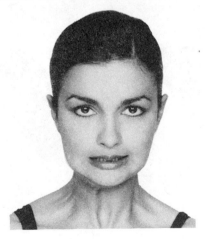

Tighten and tuck in your chin, bringing it down slightly toward your chest. Squeeze so that you can feel your neck tighten. If you are doing the exercise correctly, as you look in the mirror you will see the tendons in your neck stand out like cords. Hold for a count of 3; relax. Repeat the contraction and hold 2 more times.

After 2 or 3 weeks of regular exercising, begin building up the number of repetitions gradually but do not increase the length of the hold.

# 3. Vertical Chin Wheel

This is a popular exercise with actresses and models. And with good reason. They can't afford to have a double chin. And neither can you!

Sit up straight in a chair or on the edge of your bed with your feet flat on the floor in front of you. Hold your back erect, but try to keep your shoulders and body relaxed. Your hands should rest lightly on your thighs.

Now open your mouth as wide as it will go comfortably. Try to ignore your upper jaw, while the lower one does all the work.

Leading always with your chin, slowly stretch your lower jaw first down and then out as far as it will go; then slowly raise it. Push your chin away from you as far as you can, as in a growl, while simultaneously moving it up slowly. Keep the rest of your head motionless.

When your teeth stop you from going any farther, pull your jaw back in slowly as far as it will go and then bring it down, returning to the starting position. Think of your lower jaw as a car on a ferris wheel to help you pattern the motion.

Next do the same exercise in reverse, pulling your jaw in and up and then out and down to return to the starting position. Repeat each wheel in opposite directions 2 more times.

After 2 or 3 weeks of exercising, increase the number of repetitions gradually.

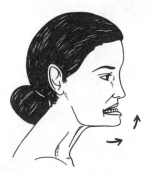 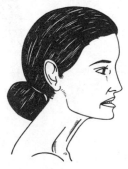

# 4. Horizontal Chin Wheel

This exercise is similar to the previous one except that the jaw motion is from side to side.

Seat yourself comfortably with erect posture, as in the previous exercise. Pick a spot to help you concentrate. The idea here is to make a circle. Push your lower jaw forward as far as it will go. Now slowly swing your jaw out and around to the left. When you've gone as far as you can go, slowly pull your jaw in, around, and back. Keeping your chin as far as you can hold it, continue the circle by moving your jaw toward the right. When you've reached the point on the right to which you can comfortably move, push out again, swinging your jaw around until it juts out straight in front of you in the starting position. Practice the same pattern of motion in the opposite direction. Repeat left and right horizontal wheels once more.

After 2 or 3 weeks of regular exercising, when this movement becomes more natural and feels less stressful, increase the number of repetitions gradually.

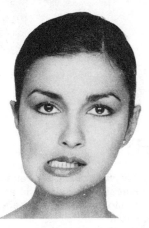

# 5. The Exorcist

Here is an easy way to exorcise those crepey chicken-skin folds that can ruin a perfectly lovely neckline. This stretch also helps to banish a double chin.

Sit straight in a chair with your feet planted flat on the ground in front of you. Try to keep your shoulders dropped and the lower part of your body relaxed. Be sure your posture is erect, with your back straight and your head level.

First pull your chin back and in. Now slowly and smoothly turn your head to the left as far as it will go comfortably without moving your trunk. When your head is twisted around as far as you think it can go, stretch your neck a bit higher (but do not stick out your chin) and then gently try to rotate your head a little farther to the left. Hold for a count of 3. Slowly return to the starting position. Practice the same movement, twisting your head to the right. Repeat the head twists to the left and right 2 more times.

Be sure that all these motions are slow and smooth. Do not jerk your neck or try to force your head around farther than it will turn naturally, or you could hurt yourself. Slow, gentle movements will tone the muscles and gradually give you a fuller range of motion. You will be surprised at your progress in just a few weeks.

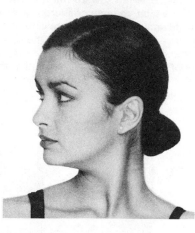

# PRETTY BABY

The rosebud lips of youth are not just a poetic metaphor. A firm, supple mouth, capable of the subtlest expressions, is an important component of beauty. The expression about your mouth is usually a good indicator of your general mood and muscle tone.

Sagging corners, rubbery lips, lack of good muscle control around the mouth can distort the contours of an otherwise attractive, young-looking face. The exercises that follow will help to prevent this by toning and tightening the muscles around the mouth and lips.

Because they are constructed to serve important physical functions, the mouth and lips are controlled by muscles that are relatively easy to exercise. Though we use these muscles every day in ordinary actions and expressions, we don't always use them to their fullest strength or range of motion. Slurred or mumbled speech, minimal use of facial expressions, and dental problems are all factors that can interfere with their use.

If you have a severe problem with your bite, it can affect your entire lower face. You might in this instance consider consulting a dentist or doctor.

# 6. Going to the Dickens

There is nothing new about understanding the importance of facial carriage. In 1857, in his novel *Little Dorrit*, Charles Dickens created a character named Mrs. General, a formidable governess who repeatedly admonished her charges to practice the proper facial expressions. "The word Papa . . . gives a pretty form to the lips," Mrs. General insisted. "Papa, potatoes, poultry, prunes and prism are all very good words for the lips: especially prunes and prism."

We now know that the heroine of the novel, Little Dorrit, should have listened to Mrs. General. There are physical therapy manuals that recommend just such exercises. The governess's "prunes and prisms" are excellent for toning the orbicularis oris, the muscle that rings the mouth and lips. Try saying these words and see what they do for *your* ruby reds.

Purse your lips together firmly. With an exaggerated effort on each syllable, repeat the words *papa, potatoes, poultry, prunes*, and *prism* in sequence 10 times. Each time you pronounce a "p" sound, press your lips together as hard as you can. As you finish the syllable, there should be a forced exhalation of breath. Exaggerate the pucker also wherever appropriate. Pronounce each word clearly and distinctly.

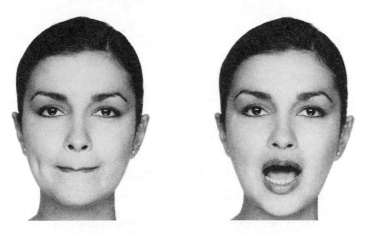

# 7. The Shirley Temple Pout

In her early films, Shirley Temple immortalized the pout. She had exactly the right gesture, thrusting out her lower lip and dimpling that adorable chin. She was much too young to worry about it at the time, but that petulant expression was just what she needed to keep her chin firm and to prevent sagging at the corners of the mouth.

If you must, let yourself feel sad or petulant for a moment, just to get the right expression. But then remember how happy you will feel when you look in the mirror after several weeks of practicing your facial exercises!

Pull your lower lip up and out, so that the soft inside of your lip is visible. Your chin will move up and in and will probably look dimpled. Push out the pout and hold it for a count of 3; relax. Repeat 2 more times.

After 2 or 3 weeks of exercising, increase the number of repetitions gradually.

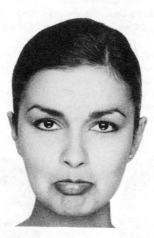

# 8. The Wolf Whistle

If it's been awhile since you've heard a wolf whistle, start practicing them yourself. Soon they'll be aimed in your direction every time you walk down the street. This is wonderful for the cheek muscles under the cheekbone.

Pucker your lips and whistle for 5 seconds. Wolf whistles are fine, but if you can handle a tune, you'll probably find it more interesting. If you can't whistle, just pucker your lips, tighten them, and blow. Relax after 5 seconds. Repeat 2 more times.

After 2 or 3 weeks, you can increase the benefits of this exercise by whistling for longer periods of time and / or by increasing the number of repetitions.

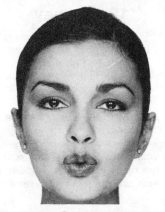

# 9. The Straightaway

Jack Benny was a master of this expression. If you are a Gilda Radner fan, you'll recognize it as an Emily Littella special. If neither of these rings a bell, think of it as a deadpan grin, a suppressed smile in which the corners of the mouth are pulled straight back but not up. This is an important exercise for toning the corners of the mouth. It also helps to support sagging jowls.

It is best to practice this exercise with your lips together, but some people find it easier to do with their mouths slightly open. Pull the corners of your mouth back toward the sides of your head, but don't allow yourself to raise your cheeks into a smile. Check in the mirror to be sure you keep your mouth in as straight a line as possible. Tighten your lip and cheek muscles and hold for a count of 3, then relax. Repeat 2 more times.

After 2 or 3 weeks of exercising, increase the number of repetitions gradually.

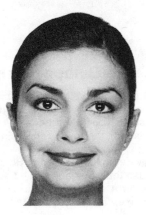

# 10. Phooey

Saying "phooey" isn't just a lot of hooey. Working that upper lip will tone and tighten the tissues between your lip and your nose, where that fine accordion pleating often appears first on delicate skin. If they're allowed to develop, those wrinkles above the lip can spoil the most winsome cupid's bow.

Pronounce the word *phooey*. Put the emphasis on the first syllable. Draw it out and exaggerate the sound, stretching your upper lip out and up. This motion will also exercise muscles over the bridge and along the sides of the nose. Think of showing your gums over your top front teeth as you say it. Or try to touch your lip to the tip of your nose. Repeat 4 more times.

After 2 or 3 weeks, increase the number of repetitions gradually.

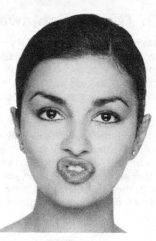

# 11. The Disappearing Act

It would be nice if we could make lines and wrinkles disappear with a snap of our fingers. Unfortunately, it's not as easy as that. But you can work diligently to keep your face as young and healthy-looking as nature intended. Here is one final exercise for the lower face—lips, mouth, jowls, chin.

Pull in your lips gently between your teeth. Holding them together, tighten from the sides as well, so that they are pursed as hard as they can be and almost disappear. Hold for a count of 3; relax. Repeat 2 more times.

After 2 or 3 weeks of exercising, increase the number of repetitions gradually.

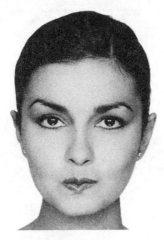

# CHEEK TO CHEEK

When you're talking about sagging and bagging, this central area of the face is where a lot of the weight comes from. For a look of freshness and youthful expressiveness, it is particularly important to exercise these muscles over the cheeks and around the nose.

A properly used, toned muscle holds its shape. Toning will help to prevent both puffiness and that unhealthy, sunken look.

Because of the way many of these muscles intersect, you'll find that by exercising your cheeks, jaw, and nasal areas, you will often be working your lips and temples as well—an added bonus!

A mirror will help you with most of these facial maneuvers. Don't hold back or skip an exercise because you think it makes you look silly. Remember, each pose is held only for a few moments. No one is watching. And the ultimate benefits were designed to keep you happy for a long time.

## 12. Facial Twist

If you think you look silly doing this exercise, wait until you see what it does for your face. It will tone your cheeks as well as the corners of your mouth and that delicate area under the eye.

Sit comfortably with your back straight and your head level. Without moving your head, bring your eyes diagonally up and to the right. You'll feel your cheek and temple muscles lift slightly. Now screw up your mouth, keeping your lips together, to follow your eyes. Tighten the muscles in a strong contraction. Hold for a count of 3; relax. Follow the same motions in exercising your left side. Repeat right and left facial twists 2 more times.

After 2 or 3 weeks of exercising, increase the number of repetitions gradually.

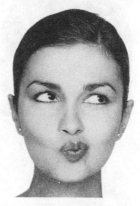

# 13. Balloon Twist

By creating tension from the inside, this exercise helps to tighten and develop the cheek muscles. It will also work on crinkles around the mouth and help tone sagging jowls.

With your lips together, screw up your mouth and twist it around to the left, as you did in the previous exercise. Now force air into your right cheek so that it balloons out tightly. Push the inside of your cheek back against the pressure of the air toward the teeth. Hold to a count of 3; relax.

Twist your mouth around to the right and inflate your left cheek with air. Push and hold to a count of 3; relax. Repeat left and right twists and holds 2 more times.

After exercising for 2 or 3 weeks, increase the number of repetitions gradually.

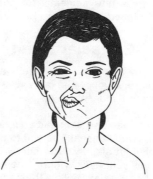

# 14. Nasal Lift

Many facial muscles are small and difficult to develop. This exercise works on the thin muscles at the side of the nose and the round "apple" area of the cheek. Both need tightening to prevent sagging and wrinkling. This exercise also tones the area between the nose and the mouth, where laugh lines tend to form.

Place your right index finger lightly at the bottom corner of your nose, just outside your right nostril. The light pressure of this finger will help you to feel the motion of the muscles.

Dilate your right nostril, flaring it up and out as far as you can. When you do this, you will feel your finger rise as your cheek moves up also. If you are working with a mirror, you will see your mouth move to the side as well, but do not twist it intentionally. Try to let the specific muscles in your nose and cheek do the work. Hold the lift to a count of 3; relax. Practice the same motion on the left side, using your left index finger as a guide. Repeat right and left lifts 2 more times.

After exercising for 2 or 3 weeks, increase the number of repetitions gradually.

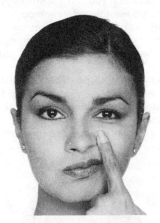

# 15. The Sleek Cheek

This simple exercise can be beneficial in several ways. By toning the cheek muscles, it can help to prevent sagging jowls. By developing those muscles, it can help to fill out sunken cheeks. And by tightening the tissues, it may minimize wrinkling over the cheek area.

With your mouth closed, suck in your cheeks. Pull the flesh in over your back molars. Your teeth will move wider apart as you pull in farther, but keep your lips, which will look puckered, together. Hold to a count of 5; relax. Repeat 2 more times.

After 2 or 3 weeks of exercising, increase the length of the hold and the number of repetitions gradually.

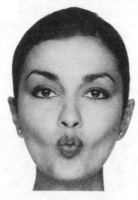

# 16. The Eraser

Don't you wish you could just rub out those fragile smile lines drooping from the side of your nose down toward your mouth? They can be positively heartbreaking when they first occur. Well, you shouldn't stop smiling, and looking your best will make you smile all the more; so practice this exercise, which will smooth out those lines and tighten the tissues underneath.

Dilate your nostrils as widely as possible. Flare them out at the edges rather than scrunching up your nose. Put your lips together and draw the corners of your mouth downward as far as possible. Hold to a count of 3; relax. Repeat 2 more times.

After 2 or 3 weeks of exercising, increase the number of repetitions gradually.

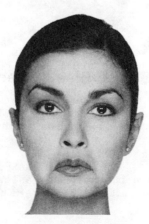

## 17. Tight Clench

A tight, well-defined jawline gives a youthful look to any face. We use our jaw muscles whenever we eat, but most of us tend to chew our food on a preferred side. This can leave the other side flaccid and poorly toned. Because the muscles of mastication, as they are called, are so powerful, unbalanced development can lead to an uneven appearance of the jawline or even throw off the balance of the entire face.

If you have problems with your bite that interfere with your ability to clench your teeth properly, you might consider consulting an orthodontist who specializes in such problems. More and more adults are doing so. If your bite is relatively normal, this simple exercise should be enough. Surprisingly, it will tighten the temple area as well.

Place your teeth comfortably together and clench your jaw as hard as you can. Concentrate your strength on your molars in back. Hold to a count of 3; relax. Repeat 2 more times.

After 2 or 3 weeks of exericising, increase the number of repetitions gradually.

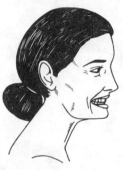

# THE EYES HAVE IT

All the attention, that is. Ask someone what facial feature they notice first, and nine out of ten times it's the eyes. They are a beautiful woman's greatest asset. But just try batting lashes surrounded by crepe-paper skin, droopy lizard lids, and puffy bags. You're sure to strike out! That's why it's particularly important to prevent wrinkling and sagging around the eyes for as long as possible.

The eye area is very difficult to deal with. The tissues are extremely delicate, and there are not a lot of muscles to work with. But the following exercises will help. (So will Exercises 12, 17, 23, and 24.) A good eye cream can also prevent wrinkles for awhile.

As a last resort, of course, it is reassuring to remember that cosmetic plastic surgery can deal nicely with droopy eyelids in an operation called blepharoplasty, which usually requires only two days in the hospital.

# 18. The Round-the-Clock Rotation

This exercise takes most people about half a minute. It is excellent for the muscles around the eyeball. If you wear contact lenses, remove them to prevent slippage.

Imagine the face of a clock drawn around your head with twelve o'clock directly above your head, three o'clock next to your right ear, six o'clock below your chin, and nine o'clock next to your left ear. Keeping your head level, look up as high as you can to the twelve o'clock position. Slowly rotate your eyes clockwise as if tracing the minutes all the way around. After you've returned to the twelve o'clock position, relax for a moment and then repeat the exercise in a counterclockwise direction.

Some people find it easier to follow this exercise if they use a finger as a sort of minute-hand guide. Use your right index finger to trace twelve through six o'clock and your left index finger for six back up to twelve.

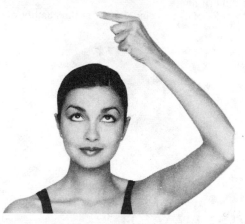

# 19. Upper Lid Lift

There is not much you can do for crepey eyelids, short of plastic surgery. But here is an exercise that will help forestall wrinkles on that delicate skin as long as possible. Be sure you follow the instructions carefully and do not place any pressure on your eyeball.

Close your eyes lightly. Place your thumb and index fingers gently at the outside corners of your eye socket, so that your index finger rests on the edge of the bone and the tip of the finger anchors your upper eyelid. Again, do not put any pressure on the eyeball. Now slowly pull your upper lid up so that you open your eyes wide. Use the leverage of your fingers to create a slight resistance, but do not pull the lids down with your fingers or you will stretch the skin. Repeat 2 more times.

After 2 or 3 weeks of exercising, increase the number of repetitions.

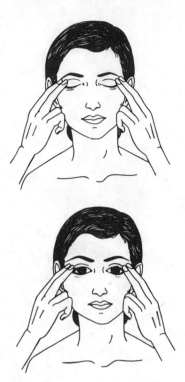

# 20. Lower Lid Lift—Bagging It

Bags under the eyes are most unattractive. They age the face and often look unhealthy. To help minimize bagging, be sure you get enough sleep at night. Try an extra pillow to relieve some of the puffiness. This exercise to tone the lower eyelid will firm up the tissues under the eye and help prevent bagging and sagging.

Open your eyes wide. Hold your upper lids open by lightly pinning your upper lashes against the bone of the eye socket with the length of your index finger. There should be no pressure on your eyeball at all.

Now try to close your eyes by pulling up the lower lids as high as you can. When you can go no farther, release the pressure on the lashes so that your eyes close naturally. Repeat 2 more times.

After 2 or 3 weeks of exercising, increase the number of repetitions gradually.

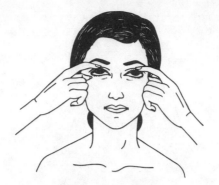

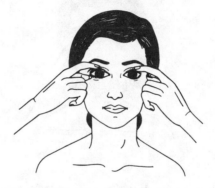

# 21. The Big Squeeze

Crow's-feet, those fine radiating lines at the outside edge of the eye, are often the first signs of age to appear in an otherwise youthful face.

About all you can do for the eye area, aside from shielding it from harmful sun rays and religiously applying a good moisturizing cream, is to practice contractions that will tone the area to keep it as tight and firm as possible. This exercise is for the orbicularis oculi, the muscle that encircles the eye socket.

Close your right eye and squeeze it tightly. Hold to a count of 3; relax. Close your left eye and squeeze it shut. Hold the contraction to a count of 3; relax. Repeat left and right squeezes 2 more times.

Some people have difficulty closing one eye at a time. If you are one of them, simply close both your eyes together and squeeze. Hold to a count of 3; open your eyes and relax. Repeat 2 more times.

After exercising for 2 or 3 weeks, increase the number of repetitions gradually.

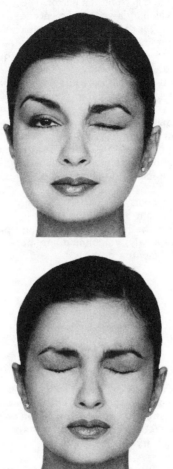

# MIRROR, MIRROR

This final section is designed to finish off your facial exercise program with a feeling of total tightness—your all-natural face-lift. All of these exercises should be performed in front of a mirror. They are more subtle than the others and involve developing a sense of awareness of certain muscles that are difficult to control. Consequently, it may take you a bit more time to master them. Since the first three exercises involve little change of facial expression, precise line drawings with arrows for guidance have been included. Be patient and work diligently.

By now you must feel as if your face has had quite a workout. It has! After you finish this final group of exercises, complete the program with the following:

1. Lie down and wrap your face in a warm—not hot—towel. Relax and try to think pleasant thoughts for at least 3 minutes. You want to give those muscles a chance to rest after that vigorous workout.
2. Give your face a thorough cleansing. Stimulate the skin gently with your fingertips or a specially designed mildly dermabrasive pad as you wash.
3. Apply a mild astringent.
4. Cover your face with a good moisturizer.
5. Take a long look in the mirror. I hope you are pleased. If you practice your exercises regularly, you should see more and more improvement as the weeks and months go by.

# 22. Scalp Lift

When we're tired, our shoulders tend to droop, our bodies to sag. Have you ever caught yourself and used your energy to pull yourself up, correct your posture, stand up straight? Try the same idea on your face. When we're tired or depressed, our facial muscles tend to sag too. Aging has a similar effect. For an instant lift, try the following:

Standing in front of a mirror to be sure that your form is correct, open your eyes wide, lift your eyebrows, and pull back your forehead and scalp as far as you can. At the same time, try to pull your scalp down at the back of your head (tightening your neck and shoulders can help you to achieve this sensation at first). Be sure that you do *not* wrinkle your forehead as you do this exercise. Hold the lift for a count of 3; relax. Repeat 2 more times.

After 2 or 3 weeks of exercising, increase the number of repetitions gradually.

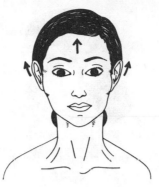

# 23. Howdy Doody

If you're old enough to remember Howdy, you're ready for this exercise. It's a total upper facial lift that's particularly effective around the eyes. It looks marvelous, but it can take some time to become aware of these seldom-used muscles and to learn to control them. Use your mirror to help.

Rather than just an exercise, think of this movement as a pose to strike any time you want to look your best.

The intent of this exercise is to tighten the temporalis muscles, the muscles that extend from your temples back over the sides of your head, and the small muscles in front of your ears. The best way to perform this is to try and wiggle your ears, like Howdy, by pulling your scalp back and up. Placing your index fingers lightly on the soft skin in front of your ears may help you to develop an awareness of this muscle and to feel it tighten. Raising the outside edges of your eyebrows and thinking of pulling them back toward your ears will also help. There should be little or no wrinkling of your forehead.

Practiced properly, you will experience a definite tightening sensation throughout the entire upper face, primarily in the temple area, but there will be little change of expression.

This is a difficult pose to hold at first; so in the beginning, simply practice a few repetitions. Once you have more control and the exercise does not feel stressful, begin holding the pose longer as well as increasing the number of repetitions.

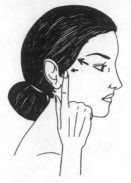

# 24. Total Temple Toner

This is a marvelous exercise that will really give you a workout. It will tighten the area around the temple, helping to smooth out crinkly crow's feet at the outside corners of the eye and over the cheekbone. It is also excellent for tightening the soft fleshy area under the chin.

Tighten your scalp as much as you can by pulling it both backward and to the sides, as illustrated in Exercises 22 and 23. Now press your tongue flat up against the roof of your mouth. Concentrate on pushing the middle and back of your tongue against the hard palate. Hold for a count of 3; release. Repeat 2 more times.

This is a strenuous contraction, so don't overdo it. After you have been exercising for a number of weeks and it no longer feels stressful, increase the number of repetitions gradually.

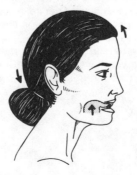

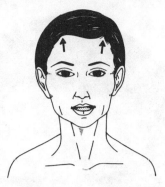

# 25. Pretty Face

This is the best exercise of all, and it has nothing to do with muscle development directly. Now that you've been working with your face, you should feel a much greater sense of mobility and control. This will increase dramatically as you exercise regularly over a period of months. Use it to your advantage.

Take a good look at your face in the mirror. Learn to see your assets as well as your problem spots. Experiment with different expressions. Your "natural" expression at rest, largely a matter of habit, may not be the most flattering to you. Observe the change when you tighten your scalp, raise your eyebrows, move your jaw.

Is your smile the most beguiling you can make it? There are many different ways to smile. Try them out.

Become aware of your facial carriage. Confidence and poise are important components of beauty. Learn to control your facial muscles so that others see you as you choose to be seen.

Most of all, think pretty! If *you* like the way you look, others will too.

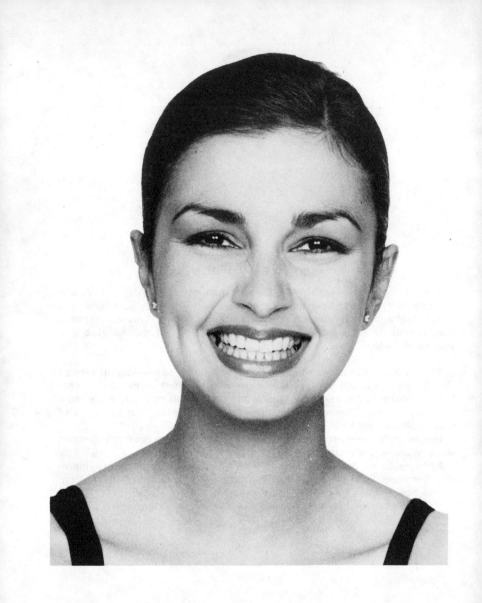